THYROID-HEALING RECIPES COOKBOOK FOR HORMONE BALANCE

Nourishing Your Body, Restoring Your Vitality

LAUREN WILLS

CONTENTS

INTRODUCTION

Welcome to "Thyroid-Healing Recipes for Hormone Balance: Nourishing Your Body, Restoring Your Vitality." This cookbook is a culinary journey designed to empower you with delicious and health-conscious recipes aimed at promoting thyroid health and hormonal balance.

The thyroid gland, a small but mighty butterfly-shaped organ in our neck, plays a significant role in regulating our metabolism and overall well-being. When our thyroid is out of balance, it can affect various aspects of our lives, from energy levels and mood to weight management and immune function.

Living with thyroid imbalances, whether it's hypothyroidism or hyperthyroidism, can be challenging, but we believe that the foods we consume can make a significant difference in our journey toward healing and vitality. The recipes in this cookbook are thoughtfully crafted to incorporate ingredients known to support thyroid health and hormonal equilibrium.

Inside these pages, you'll discover a diverse array of dishes, from vibrant salads and hearty mains to revitalizing smoothies and nourishing sides. Each recipe is designed not only to tantalize your taste buds but also to provide essential nutrients that can contribute to a healthier thyroid.

We understand that maintaining a balanced diet can be a crucial part of managing thyroid conditions, so we've made it our mission to create recipes that are not only beneficial but also enjoyable for everyone at the table. Whether you're cooking for yourself or your loved ones, these recipes are designed to be both nourishing and delicious.

Our hope is that these recipes will not only support your journey to thyroid health but also make mealtime a delightful and positive experience. We encourage you to explore, experiment, and savor each dish as you embark on your path toward hormone balance and overall vitality.

Remember, healing can be a flavorful and fulfilling journey. Let's cook our way to a healthier thyroid and a more vibrant life together.

THYROID-HEALING RECIPES

Recipe 1: Hormone-Balancing Breakfast Smoothie

Prep Time: 5 minutes

Ingredients:

- 1 ripe banana
- 1/2 cup Greek yogurt
- 1/2 cup spinach leaves
- 1/4 cup blueberries
- 1 tablespoon flaxseeds
- 1/2 cup almond milk

Directions:

1. Place all ingredients in a blender.
2. Blend until smooth.
3. Pour into a glass and enjoy!

Nutritional Value: Calories: 250 | Protein: 12g | Carbohydrates: 40g | Fiber: 7g | Fat: 6g

Recipe 2: Quinoa and Roasted Veggie Bowl

Prep Time: 30 minutes

Ingredients:

- 1 cup quinoa
- 2 cups mixed vegetables (bell peppers, broccoli, carrots)

- 2 tablespoons olive oil

- 1 teaspoon cumin

- 1/2 teaspoon paprika

- Salt and pepper to taste

Directions:

1. Cook quinoa according to package instructions.

2. Toss mixed vegetables with olive oil, cumin, paprika, salt, and pepper.

3. Roast at 400°F (200°C) for 20 minutes.

4. Serve roasted veggies over cooked quinoa.

Nutritional Value: Calories: 350 | Protein: 8g | Carbohydrates: 56g | Fiber: 9g | Fat: 12g

Recipe 3: Thyroid-Boosting Salmon Salad

Prep Time: 15 minutes

Ingredients:

- 2 cups mixed greens

- 4 oz grilled salmon

- 1/4 cup cherry tomatoes

- 1/4 cup cucumber, sliced

- 1/4 cup red onion, thinly sliced

- 2 tablespoons balsamic vinaigrette

Directions:

1. Arrange mixed greens on a plate.

2. Top with grilled salmon, cherry tomatoes, cucumber, and red onion.

3. Drizzle with balsamic vinaigrette.

Nutritional Value: Calories: 300 | Protein: 25g | Carbohydrates: 10g | Fiber: 3g | Fat: 18g

Recipe 4: Hormone-Healing Lentil Soup

Prep Time: 45 minutes

Ingredients:

- 1 cup dried green lentils
- 1 onion, chopped
- 2 carrots, diced
- 2 celery stalks, chopped
- 2 cloves garlic, minced
- 1 teaspoon turmeric
- 1/2 teaspoon cumin
- 4 cups vegetable broth
- Salt and pepper to taste

Directions:

1. In a large pot, sauté onion, carrots, celery, and garlic until softened.

2. Add lentils, turmeric, and cumin. Stir for 1-2 minutes.

3. Pour in vegetable broth and simmer for 30-35 minutes.

4. Season with salt and pepper.

Nutritional Value: Calories: 250 | Protein: 15g | Carbohydrates: 45g | Fiber: 15g | Fat: 1g

Recipe 5: Berry Chia Pudding

Prep Time: 10 minutes (+ 4 hours refrigeration)
Ingredients:

- 2 tablespoons chia seeds
- 1/2 cup almond milk
- 1/2 cup mixed berries (strawberries, blueberries, raspberries)
- 1 teaspoon honey (optional)

Directions:

1. Mix chia seeds and almond milk in a jar.
2. Refrigerate for at least 4 hours or overnight.
3. Layer chia pudding with mixed berries.
4. Drizzle with honey if desired.

Nutritional Value: Calories: 180 | Protein: 4g | Carbohydrates: 23g | Fiber: 10g | Fat: 8g

Recipe 6: Sweet Potato and Chickpea Curry

Prep Time: 40 minutes

Ingredients:

- 2 sweet potatoes, diced
- 1 can chickpeas, drained and rinsed
- 1 onion, chopped

- 2 cloves garlic, minced
- 1 can diced tomatoes
- 1 can coconut milk
- 2 tablespoons curry powder
- Salt and pepper to taste

Directions:

1. In a large pot, sauté onion and garlic until fragrant.
2. Add sweet potatoes, chickpeas, diced tomatoes, coconut milk, and curry powder.
3. Simmer for 25-30 minutes until sweet potatoes are tender.
4. Season with salt and pepper.

Nutritional Value: Calories: 350 | Protein: 9g | Carbohydrates: 48g | Fiber: 10g | Fat: 16g

Recipe 7: Spinach and Mushroom Omelette

Prep Time: 15 minutes

Ingredients:

- 2 eggs
- 1/4 cup spinach leaves, chopped
- 1/4 cup mushrooms, sliced
- 2 tablespoons grated Parmesan cheese
- Salt and pepper to taste
- Cooking spray

Directions:

1. Whisk eggs in a bowl and season with salt and pepper.

2. Heat a non-stick skillet over medium heat, coat with cooking spray.

3. Pour whisked eggs into the skillet.

4. Add spinach, mushrooms, and Parmesan cheese on one half.

5. Fold the other half over the filling.

6. Cook until set, then flip and cook the other side.

Nutritional Value: Calories: 220 | Protein: 16g | Carbohydrates: 4g | Fiber: 1g | Fat: 16g

Recipe 8: Avocado and Tomato Salad

Prep Time: 10 minutes

Ingredients:

- 1 ripe avocado, diced

- 1 cup cherry tomatoes, halved

- 1/4 cup red onion, finely chopped

- 2 tablespoons fresh cilantro, chopped

- Juice of 1 lime

- Salt and pepper to taste

Directions:

1. In a bowl, combine diced avocado, cherry tomatoes, red onion, and cilantro.

2. Drizzle with lime juice and season with salt and pepper.

Nutritional Value: Calories: 180 | Protein: 2g | Carbohydrates: 12g | Fiber: 6g | Fat: 15g

Recipe 9: Baked Salmon with Asparagus

Prep Time: 25 minutes

Ingredients:

- 4 salmon fillets
- 1 bunch asparagus
- 2 cloves garlic, minced
- 2 tablespoons olive oil
- 1 lemon, sliced
- Salt and pepper to taste

Directions:

1. Preheat oven to 375°F (190°C).
2. Place salmon fillets and asparagus on a baking sheet.
3. Drizzle with olive oil, sprinkle minced garlic, and season with salt and pepper.
4. Top with lemon slices.
5. Bake for 15-20 minutes or until salmon flakes easily.

Nutritional Value: Calories: 320 | Protein: 35g | Carbohydrates: 7g | Fiber: 3g | Fat: 18g

Recipe 10: Hormone-Balancing Berry Parfait

Prep Time: 10 minutes

Ingredients:

- 1 cup Greek yogurt

- 1/2 cup mixed berries (strawberries, blueberries, raspberries)

- 2 tablespoons honey

- 1/4 cup granola

Directions:

1. Layer Greek yogurt, mixed berries, honey, and granola in a glass.

2. Repeat the layers.

3. Finish with a drizzle of honey on top.

Nutritional Value: Calories: 280 | Protein: 15g | Carbohydrates: 42g | Fiber: 4g | Fat: 6g

Recipe 11: Quinoa-Stuffed Bell Peppers

Prep Time: 45 minutes

Ingredients:

- 4 bell peppers, halved and seeded

- 1 cup cooked quinoa

- 1 cup black beans, drained and rinsed

- 1 cup corn kernels

- 1 cup diced tomatoes

- 1 teaspoon chili powder

- 1/2 cup shredded cheddar cheese (optional)

- Salt and pepper to taste

Directions:

1. Preheat oven to 375°F (190°C).

2. In a bowl, mix quinoa, black beans, corn, diced tomatoes, and chili powder. Season with salt and pepper.

3. Stuff each bell pepper half with the quinoa mixture.

4. Bake for 25-30 minutes.

5. Sprinkle with cheddar cheese if desired, and bake for an additional 5 minutes until cheese melts.

Nutritional Value: Calories: 280 | Protein: 11g | Carbohydrates: 50g | Fiber: 10g | Fat: 5g

Recipe 12: Cucumber and Dill Salad

Prep Time: 10 minutes

Ingredients:

- 2 cucumbers, thinly sliced

- 1/4 cup plain yogurt

- 2 tablespoons fresh dill, chopped

- 1 tablespoon lemon juice

- Salt and pepper to taste

Directions:

1. In a bowl, combine cucumber slices, plain yogurt, fresh dill, and lemon juice.

2. Season with salt and pepper.

Nutritional Value: Calories: 60 | Protein: 2g | Carbohydrates: 10g | Fiber: 2g | Fat: 2g

Recipe 13: Sautéed Brussels Sprouts with Almonds

Prep Time: 20 minutes

Ingredients:

- 1 pound Brussels sprouts, trimmed and halved

- 2 tablespoons olive oil

- 1/4 cup slivered almonds

- 2 cloves garlic, minced

- Salt and pepper to taste

Directions:

1. Heat olive oil in a skillet over medium heat.

2. Add Brussels sprouts and sauté until tender and slightly browned.

3. Stir in slivered almonds and minced garlic, cook for another 2 minutes.

4. Season with salt and pepper.

Nutritional Value: Calories: 180 | Protein: 6g | Carbohydrates: 12g | Fiber: 4g | Fat: 14g

Recipe 14: Broccoli and Spinach Soup

Prep Time: 30 minutes

Ingredients:

- 2 cups broccoli florets
- 2 cups spinach leaves
- 1 onion, chopped
- 2 cloves garlic, minced
- 4 cups vegetable broth
- 1/2 cup plain yogurt (optional)
- Salt and pepper to taste

Directions:

1. In a large pot, sauté onion and garlic until softened.
2. Add broccoli florets and spinach leaves. Sauté for 5 minutes.
3. Pour in vegetable broth and simmer for 20 minutes.
4. Blend until smooth. Stir in plain yogurt if desired.
5. Season with salt and pepper.

Nutritional Value: Calories: 150 | Protein: 7g | Carbohydrates: 20g | Fiber: 6g | Fat: 5g

Recipe 15: Grilled Chicken with Lemon-Herb Marinade

Prep Time: 20 minutes

Ingredients:

- 4 boneless, skinless chicken breasts

- Juice of 2 lemons

- 2 tablespoons olive oil

- 2 cloves garlic, minced

- 1 teaspoon dried thyme

- 1 teaspoon dried rosemary

- Salt and pepper to taste

Directions:

1. In a bowl, mix lemon juice, olive oil, minced garlic, thyme, rosemary, salt, and pepper.

2. Marinate chicken breasts in the mixture for at least 15 minutes.

3. Grill chicken until cooked through, about 6-8 minutes per side.

Nutritional Value: Calories: 280 | Protein: 40g | Carbohydrates: 3g | Fiber: 1g | Fat: 11g

Recipe 16: Roasted Beet and Citrus Salad

Prep Time: 40 minutes

Ingredients:

- 4 beets, peeled and diced

- 2 oranges, peeled and segmented

- 1 grapefruit, peeled and segmented

- 1/4 cup red onion, thinly sliced

- 2 tablespoons fresh mint leaves, chopped

- 2 tablespoons balsamic vinegar

- 2 tablespoons olive oil

- Salt and pepper to taste

Directions:

1. Preheat oven to 400°F (200°C).

2. Toss diced beets with olive oil and roast for 30-35 minutes until tender.

3. In a bowl, combine roasted beets, orange segments, grapefruit segments, red onion, and fresh mint.

4. Drizzle with balsamic vinegar, and season with salt and pepper.

Nutritional Value: Calories: 190 | Protein: 3g | Carbohydrates: 30g | Fiber: 6g | Fat: 8g

Recipe 17: Butternut Squash and Apple Soup

Prep Time: 45 minutes

Ingredients:

- 2 cups butternut squash, diced

- 2 apples, peeled, cored, and diced

- 1 onion, chopped

- 2 cloves garlic, minced

- 4 cups vegetable broth

- 1/2 cup coconut milk (optional)

- 1 teaspoon cinnamon

- Salt and pepper to taste

Directions:

1. In a large pot, sauté onion and garlic until softened.

2. Add butternut squash and apples, sauté for 5 minutes.

3. Pour in vegetable broth and simmer for 30 minutes.

4. Blend until smooth. Stir in coconut milk and cinnamon if desired.

5. Season with salt and pepper.

Nutritional Value: Calories: 200 | Protein: 2g | Carbohydrates: 32g | Fiber: 5g | Fat: 8g

Recipe 18: Mediterranean Quinoa Salad

Prep Time: 20 minutes

Ingredients:

- 2 cups cooked quinoa

- 1 cup cherry tomatoes, halved

- 1/2 cucumber, diced

- 1/4 cup Kalamata olives, sliced

- 1/4 cup feta cheese, crumbled

- 2 tablespoons fresh parsley, chopped

- 2 tablespoons olive oil

- Juice of 1 lemon

- Salt and pepper to taste

Directions:

1. In a bowl, combine cooked quinoa, cherry tomatoes, cucumber, Kalamata olives, feta cheese, and fresh parsley.

2. Drizzle with olive oil and lemon juice.

3. Season with salt and pepper.

Nutritional Value: Calories: 280 | Protein: 8g | Carbohydrates: 32g | Fiber: 4g | Fat: 15g

Recipe 19: Ginger and Turmeric Carrot Soup

Prep Time: 35 minutes

Ingredients:

- 4 cups carrots, sliced

- 1 onion, chopped

- 2 cloves garlic, minced

- 2 teaspoons ginger, grated

- 2 teaspoons turmeric powder

- 4 cups vegetable broth

- 1/2 cup coconut milk (optional)

- Salt and pepper to taste

Directions:

1. In a large pot, sauté onion, garlic, ginger, and turmeric until fragrant.

2. Add sliced carrots and sauté for 5 minutes.

3. Pour in vegetable broth and simmer for 20-25 minutes.

4. Blend until smooth. Stir in coconut milk if desired.

5. Season with salt and pepper.

Nutritional Value: Calories: 180 | Protein: 3g | Carbohydrates: 26g | Fiber: 7g | Fat: 8g

Recipe 20: Almond-Crusted Baked Chicken

Prep Time: 30 minutes **Ingredients:**

- 4 boneless, skinless chicken breasts
- 1/2 cup almonds, finely chopped
- 1/4 cup whole wheat breadcrumbs
- 1 teaspoon paprika
- 1/2 teaspoon garlic powder
- 2 eggs, beaten
- Salt and pepper to taste

Directions:

1. Preheat oven to 375°F (190°C).

2. In a bowl, combine chopped almonds, breadcrumbs, paprika, garlic powder, salt, and pepper.

3. Dip each chicken breast in beaten eggs, then coat with the almond mixture.

4. Place coated chicken on a baking sheet.

5. Bake for 20-25 minutes until chicken is cooked through and coating is crispy.

Nutritional Value: Calories: 280 | Protein: 30g | Carbohydrates: 8g | Fiber: 3g | Fat: 15g

Recipe 21: Green Bean and Walnut Salad

Prep Time: 15 minutes

Ingredients:

- 2 cups green beans, blanched and cut into pieces
- 1/2 cup walnuts, chopped
- 1/4 cup red onion, finely chopped
- 2 tablespoons olive oil
- 1 tablespoon balsamic vinegar
- Salt and pepper to taste

Directions:

1. In a bowl, combine blanched green beans, chopped walnuts, and finely chopped red onion.
2. Drizzle with olive oil and balsamic vinegar.
3. Season with salt and pepper.

Nutritional Value: Calories: 180 | Protein: 4g | Carbohydrates: 8g | Fiber: 4g | Fat: 16g

Recipe 22: Lemon Garlic Shrimp Stir-Fry

Prep Time: 20 minutes

Ingredients:

- 1 pound large shrimp, peeled and deveined
- 2 cloves garlic, minced

- Juice of 1 lemon

- 2 tablespoons olive oil

- 1 red bell pepper, sliced

- 1 yellow bell pepper, sliced

- 1 cup broccoli florets

- Salt and pepper to taste

Directions:

1. In a bowl, marinate shrimp in minced garlic, lemon juice, olive oil, salt, and pepper for 10 minutes.

2. Heat a wok or large skillet over high heat.

3. Stir-fry bell peppers and broccoli for 2-3 minutes.

4. Add marinated shrimp and cook until they turn pink and opaque.

5. Serve immediately.

Nutritional Value: Calories: 250 | Protein: 28g | Carbohydrates: 10g | Fiber: 3g | Fat: 12g

Recipe 23: Cauliflower Rice Stir-Fry

Prep Time: 25 minutes

Ingredients:

- 1 head cauliflower, riced

- 1 cup mixed vegetables (peas, carrots, corn)

- 2 tablespoons soy sauce

- 2 cloves garlic, minced

- 1 teaspoon ginger, grated

- 2 eggs, beaten

- 2 tablespoons sesame oil

- Salt and pepper to taste

Directions:

1. In a large skillet, heat sesame oil over medium heat.

2. Add minced garlic and grated ginger, sauté for 1 minute.

3. Add mixed vegetables and cauliflower rice. Cook for 5-7 minutes.

4. Push the mixture to one side of the skillet and scramble the beaten eggs on the other side.

5. Combine everything, stir in soy sauce, salt, and pepper.

6. Cook for an additional 2 minutes.

Nutritional Value: Calories: 220 | Protein: 8g | Carbohydrates: 15g | Fiber: 6g | Fat: 14g

Recipe 24: Berry and Spinach Salad with Raspberry Vinaigrette

Prep Time: 15 minutes

Ingredients:

- 4 cups baby spinach

- 1 cup mixed berries (strawberries, blueberries, raspberries)

- 1/4 cup sliced almonds

- 2 tablespoons feta cheese, crumbled

- 1/4 cup raspberry vinaigrette dressing

Directions:

1. In a bowl, combine baby spinach, mixed berries, sliced almonds, and crumbled feta cheese.

2. Drizzle with raspberry vinaigrette dressing.

Nutritional Value: Calories: 200 | Protein: 5g | Carbohydrates: 16g | Fiber: 5g | Fat: 14g

Recipe 25: Pumpkin and Cinnamon Oatmeal

Prep Time: 15 minutes

Ingredients:

- 1 cup old-fashioned oats

- 2 cups almond milk

- 1/2 cup pumpkin puree

- 1/2 teaspoon cinnamon

- 1/4 teaspoon nutmeg

- 2 tablespoons maple syrup

- 1/4 cup chopped pecans (optional)

Directions:

1. In a saucepan, combine oats and almond milk. Cook over medium heat, stirring occasionally.

2. Stir in pumpkin puree, cinnamon, nutmeg, and maple syrup.

3. Cook until oatmeal reaches desired consistency.

4. Top with chopped pecans if desired.

Nutritional Value: Calories: 250 | Protein: 6g | Carbohydrates: 44g | Fiber: 7g | Fat: 6g

Recipe 26: Spinach and Mushroom Stuffed Chicken Breast

Prep Time: 30 minutes

Ingredients:

- 4 boneless, skinless chicken breasts

- 2 cups spinach, chopped

- 1 cup mushrooms, finely chopped

- 1/4 cup feta cheese, crumbled

- 2 cloves garlic, minced

- Salt and pepper to taste

- Olive oil for cooking

Directions:

1. In a skillet, sauté mushrooms and garlic until soft. Add spinach and cook until wilted.

2. Remove from heat and stir in feta cheese. Let it cool.

3. Cut a pocket into each chicken breast. Stuff with the spinach-mushroom mixture.

4. Season chicken with salt and pepper.

5. Heat olive oil in a pan and cook chicken until no longer pink inside.

Nutritional Value: Calories: 280 | Protein: 40g | Carbohydrates: 5g | Fiber: 2g | Fat: 10g

Recipe 27: Turmeric and Ginger Tea

Prep Time: 10 minutes

Ingredients:

- 2 cups water

- 1-inch piece of ginger, sliced

- 1 teaspoon turmeric powder

- Honey (optional)

- Lemon slice (optional)

Directions:

1. In a saucepan, bring water to a boil.

2. Add ginger slices and turmeric powder.

3. Simmer for 5-7 minutes.

4. Strain into a cup.

5. Sweeten with honey and add a lemon slice if desired.

Nutritional Value: Calories: 10 | Protein: 0g | Carbohydrates: 3g | Fiber: 1g | Fat: 0g

Recipe 28: Roasted Veggie and Quinoa Bowl

Prep Time: 40 minutes

Ingredients:

- 1 cup quinoa

- 2 cups mixed vegetables (zucchini, bell peppers, eggplant)

- 2 tablespoons olive oil

- 1 teaspoon Italian seasoning

- Salt and pepper to taste

Directions:

1. Cook quinoa according to package instructions.

2. Toss mixed vegetables with olive oil, Italian seasoning, salt, and pepper.

3. Roast at 400°F (200°C) for 20-25 minutes.

4. Serve roasted veggies over cooked quinoa.

Nutritional Value: Calories: 350 | Protein: 8g | Carbohydrates: 56g | Fiber: 9g | Fat: 12g

Recipe 29: Cauliflower and Broccoli Gratin

Prep Time: 45 minutes

Ingredients:

- 1 cauliflower, cut into florets

- 1 broccoli, cut into florets

- 2 tablespoons butter

- 2 tablespoons all-purpose flour

- 1 1/2 cups milk

- 1 cup shredded cheddar cheese

- Salt and pepper to taste

- Bread crumbs for topping

Directions:

1. Steam cauliflower and broccoli until tender.

2. In a saucepan, melt butter and stir in flour.

3. Gradually add milk, stirring constantly until thickened.

4. Stir in cheddar cheese until melted.

5. Season with salt and pepper.

6. Place steamed veggies in a baking dish, pour cheese sauce over them.

7. Top with bread crumbs.

8. Bake at 375°F (190°C) for 15-20 minutes or until golden.

Nutritional Value: Calories: 250 | Protein: 10g | Carbohydrates: 20g | Fiber: 6g | Fat: 15g

Recipe 30: Mango and Avocado Salsa

Prep Time: 15 minutes

Ingredients:

- 2 ripe mangoes, diced

- 1 ripe avocado, diced

- 1/4 cup red onion, finely chopped

- 1/4 cup fresh cilantro, chopped

- Juice of 1 lime

- Salt and pepper to taste

Directions:

1. In a bowl, combine diced mangoes, diced avocado, chopped red onion, and chopped cilantro.

2. Drizzle with lime juice.

3. Season with salt and pepper.

Nutritional Value: Calories: 150 | Protein: 2g | Carbohydrates: 26g | Fiber: 7g | Fat: 6g

Recipe 31: Garlic and Lemon Roasted Brussels Sprouts
Prep Time: 25 minutes

Ingredients:

- 1 pound Brussels sprouts, trimmed and halved

- 2 tablespoons olive oil

- 2 cloves garlic, minced

- Zest and juice of 1 lemon

- Salt and pepper to taste

Directions:

1. Preheat oven to 400°F (200°C).

2. Toss Brussels sprouts with olive oil, minced garlic, lemon zest, lemon juice, salt, and pepper.

3. Roast for 20-25 minutes or until tender and caramelized.

Nutritional Value: Calories: 120 | Protein: 4g | Carbohydrates: 14g | Fiber: 5g | Fat: 7g

Recipe 32: Hormone-Boosting Berry Smoothie Bowl

Prep Time: 10 minutes

Ingredients:

- 1 cup mixed berries (strawberries, blueberries, raspberries)

- 1/2 cup Greek yogurt

- 1/4 cup granola

- 1 tablespoon honey

- 1 tablespoon chia seeds

Directions:

1. Blend mixed berries and Greek yogurt until smooth.

2. Pour into a bowl.

3. Top with granola, drizzle with honey, and sprinkle chia seeds on top.

Nutritional Value: Calories: 250 | Protein: 12g | Carbohydrates: 40g | Fiber: 7g | Fat: 6g

Recipe 33: Lemon and Herb Grilled Tofu

Prep Time: 30 minutes **Ingredients:**

- 1 block extra-firm tofu, pressed and sliced

- Juice of 1 lemon

- 2 tablespoons olive oil

- 1 teaspoon dried basil

- 1 teaspoon dried oregano

- Salt and pepper to taste

Directions:

1. In a bowl, whisk together lemon juice, olive oil, dried basil, dried oregano, salt, and pepper.

2. Marinate tofu slices in the mixture for 15 minutes.

3. Grill tofu until lightly browned and grill marks appear.

Nutritional Value: Calories: 220 | Protein: 12g | Carbohydrates: 6g | Fiber: 2g | Fat: 16g

Recipe 34: Chickpea and Spinach Curry

Prep Time: 40 minutes **Ingredients:**

- 2 cups cooked chickpeas

- 2 cups spinach leaves

- 1 onion, chopped

- 2 cloves garlic, minced

- 1 can diced tomatoes

- 1 can coconut milk

- 2 tablespoons curry powder

- Salt and pepper to taste

Directions:

1. In a large pot, sauté onion and garlic until softened.

2. Add cooked chickpeas, spinach, diced tomatoes, coconut milk, and curry powder.

3. Simmer for 20-25 minutes.

4. Season with salt and pepper.

Nutritional Value: Calories: 350 | Protein: 12g | Carbohydrates: 45g | Fiber: 12g | Fat: 17g

Recipe 35: Berry and Almond Butter Toast

Prep Time: 5 minutes **Ingredients:**

- 2 slices whole-grain bread, toasted

- 2 tablespoons almond butter

- 1/2 cup mixed berries (strawberries, blueberries, raspberries)

- Drizzle of honey (optional)

Directions:

1. Spread almond butter evenly on toasted bread slices.

2. Top with mixed berries.

3. Drizzle with honey if desired.

Nutritional Value: Calories: 250 | Protein: 9g | Carbohydrates: 35g | Fiber: 6g | Fat: 10g

Recipe 36: Sweet Potato and Black Bean Tacos

Prep Time: 30 minutes **Ingredients:**

- 2 sweet potatoes, peeled and diced

- 1 can black beans, drained and rinsed

- 1 teaspoon chili powder

- 1/2 teaspoon cumin

- 8 small whole-wheat tortillas

- Toppings: salsa, avocado, cilantro, lime wedges

Directions:

1. Roast sweet potatoes with chili powder and cumin until tender.

2. Warm tortillas in a dry skillet.

3. Assemble tacos with roasted sweet potatoes, black beans, and desired toppings.

Nutritional Value: Calories: 280 | Protein: 9g | Carbohydrates: 54g | Fiber: 10g | Fat: 4g

Recipe 37: Cilantro-Lime Quinoa Salad

Prep Time: 20 minutes **Ingredients:**

- 1 cup cooked quinoa

- 1/4 cup fresh cilantro, chopped

- Juice of 2 limes

- 1/4 cup red bell pepper, diced

- 1/4 cup corn kernels

- 1/4 cup black beans, drained and rinsed

- Salt and pepper to taste

Directions:

1. In a bowl, mix cooked quinoa, chopped cilantro, lime juice, diced red bell pepper, corn kernels, and black beans.

2. Season with salt and pepper.

Nutritional Value: Calories: 180 | Protein: 6g | Carbohydrates: 33g | Fiber: 5g | Fat: 3g

Recipe 38: Ginger and Turmeric Roasted Carrots

Prep Time: 25 minutes **Ingredients:**

- 2 cups baby carrots

- 2 tablespoons olive oil

- 1 teaspoon ginger, grated

- 1 teaspoon turmeric powder

- Salt and pepper to taste

Directions:

1. Preheat oven to 400°F (200°C).

2. Toss baby carrots with olive oil, grated ginger, turmeric powder, salt, and pepper.

3. Roast for 20-25 minutes or until tender.

Nutritional Value: Calories: 120 | Protein: 1g | Carbohydrates: 13g | Fiber: 3g | Fat: 8g

Recipe 39: Coconut and Mango Chia Pudding

Prep Time: 10 minutes (+ 4 hours refrigeration)

Ingredients:

- 2 tablespoons chia seeds

- 1/2 cup coconut milk

- 1/2 cup diced mango

- 1 tablespoon shredded coconut

- 1 teaspoon honey (optional)

Directions:

1. Mix chia seeds and coconut milk in a jar.

2. Refrigerate for at least 4 hours or overnight.

3. Layer chia pudding with diced mango and shredded coconut.

4. Drizzle with honey if desired.

Nutritional Value: Calories: 180 | Protein: 3g | Carbohydrates: 22g | Fiber: 9g | Fat: 10g

Recipe 40: Grilled Portobello Mushrooms with Balsamic Glaze

Prep Time: 20 minutes

Ingredients:

- 4 large Portobello mushrooms

- 2 tablespoons balsamic vinegar

- 2 tablespoons olive oil

- 2 cloves garlic, minced

- Fresh thyme leaves

- Salt and pepper to taste

Directions:

1. Clean mushrooms and remove stems.

2. In a bowl, whisk balsamic vinegar, olive oil, minced garlic, fresh thyme leaves, salt, and pepper.

3. Brush mushroom caps with the mixture.

4. Grill mushrooms for 5-7 minutes per side.

5. Drizzle with remaining balsamic glaze.

Nutritional Value: Calories: 100 | Protein: 3g | Carbohydrates: 8g | Fiber: 2g | Fat: 7g

Recipe 41: Mediterranean Tuna Salad

Prep Time: 15 minutes

Ingredients:

- 2 cans tuna, drained

- 1 cucumber, diced

- 1 tomato, diced

- 1/4 cup red onion, finely chopped

- 2 tablespoons Kalamata olives, sliced

- 2 tablespoons feta cheese, crumbled

- 2 tablespoons olive oil

- Juice of 1 lemon

- Salt and pepper to taste

Directions:

2. In a bowl, combine drained tuna, diced cucumber, diced tomato, finely chopped red onion, sliced Kalamata olives, and crumbled feta cheese.

3. Drizzle with olive oil and lemon juice.

4. Season with salt and pepper.

Nutritional Value: Calories: 280 | Protein: 30g | Carbohydrates: 7g | Fiber: 2g | Fat: 15g

Recipe 42: Roasted Red Pepper and Walnut Dip

Prep Time: 15 minutes

Ingredients:

- 2 roasted red peppers, peeled and seeded

- 1/2 cup walnuts

- 2 cloves garlic

- Juice of 1 lemon

- 2 tablespoons olive oil

- Salt and pepper to taste

- Red pepper flakes (optional)

Directions:

1. In a food processor, blend roasted red peppers, walnuts, garlic, lemon juice, and olive oil until smooth.

2. Season with salt, pepper, and red pepper flakes if desired.

Nutritional Value: Calories: 200 | Protein: 4g | Carbohydrates: 7g | Fiber: 2g | Fat: 18g

Recipe 43: Miso-Glazed Eggplant

Prep Time: 30 minutes

Ingredients:

- 2 Japanese eggplants, sliced
- 2 tablespoons white miso paste
- 2 tablespoons mirin
- 2 tablespoons sake
- 1 tablespoon sugar
- 1 tablespoon sesame oil
- Sesame seeds for garnish

Directions:

1. In a bowl, whisk together white miso paste, mirin, sake, sugar, and sesame oil.

2. Brush the miso glaze on both sides of eggplant slices.

3. Grill or broil eggplant until tender and slightly caramelized.

4. Sprinkle with sesame seeds before serving.

Nutritional Value: Calories: 120 | Protein: 2g | Carbohydrates: 15g | Fiber: 4g | Fat: 6g

Recipe 44: Rainbow Quinoa Salad

Prep Time: 20 minutes

Ingredients:

- 1 cup cooked rainbow quinoa

- 1 cup cherry tomatoes, halved

- 1/2 cup cucumber, diced

- 1/2 cup red bell pepper, diced

- 1/2 cup shredded carrots

- 1/4 cup red onion, finely chopped

- 2 tablespoons fresh basil, chopped

- 2 tablespoons balsamic vinaigrette dressing

- Salt and pepper to taste

Directions:

1. In a bowl, combine cooked rainbow quinoa, halved cherry tomatoes, diced cucumber, diced red bell pepper, shredded carrots, finely chopped red onion, and chopped fresh basil.

2. Drizzle with balsamic vinaigrette dressing.

3. Season with salt and pepper.

Nutritional Value: Calories: 180 | Protein: 4g | Carbohydrates: 32g | Fiber: 4g | Fat: 4g

Recipe 45: Lemon and Herb Roasted Chicken Thighs

Prep Time: 40 minutes

Ingredients:

- 4 bone-in, skin-on chicken thighs

- Juice and zest of 1 lemon

- 2 cloves garlic, minced

- 2 tablespoons fresh rosemary, chopped

- 2 tablespoons fresh thyme, chopped

- 2 tablespoons olive oil

- Salt and pepper to taste

Directions:

1. In a bowl, mix lemon juice, lemon zest, minced garlic, chopped rosemary, chopped thyme, olive oil, salt, and pepper.

2. Marinate chicken thighs in the mixture for 20 minutes.

3. Preheat oven to 375°F (190°C).

4. Place chicken thighs on a baking sheet and roast for 30-35 minutes or until cooked through.

Nutritional Value: Calories: 320 | Protein: 24g | Carbohydrates: 2g | Fiber: 1g | Fat: 24g

Recipe 46: Cucumber and Mint Infused Water

Prep Time: 5 minutes (+ 2 hours infusing time)
Ingredients:

- 1 cucumber, thinly sliced

- 10-12 fresh mint leaves

- 8 cups water

- Ice cubes (optional)

Directions:

1. In a pitcher, combine cucumber slices and fresh mint leaves.

2. Add water and stir.

3. Refrigerate for at least 2 hours to infuse flavors.

4. Serve over ice cubes if desired.

Nutritional Value: Calories: 0 | Protein: 0g | Carbohydrates: 0g | Fiber: 0g | Fat: 0g

Recipe 47: Zucchini Noodles with Pesto

Prep Time: 20 minutes

Ingredients:

- 2 medium zucchinis, spiralized into noodles

- 1/2 cup basil leaves

- 1/4 cup pine nuts

- 1/4 cup grated Parmesan cheese

- 2 cloves garlic

- 1/4 cup olive oil

- Juice of 1 lemon

- Salt and pepper to taste

Directions:

1. In a food processor, blend basil leaves, pine nuts, grated Parmesan cheese, garlic, olive oil, lemon juice, salt, and pepper until smooth.

2. Toss zucchini noodles with pesto sauce.

3. Serve chilled.

Nutritional Value: Calories: 280 | Protein: 5g | Carbohydrates: 8g | Fiber: 2g | Fat: 26g

Recipe 48: Baked Cod with Lemon and Dill

Prep Time: 25 minutes

Ingredients:

- 4 cod fillets

- Juice of 1 lemon

- 2 tablespoons olive oil

- 2 cloves garlic, minced

- 2 teaspoons dried dill

- Salt and pepper to taste

- Lemon wedges for garnish

Directions:

1. Preheat oven to 375°F (190°C).

2. Place cod fillets in a baking dish.

3. Mix lemon juice, olive oil, minced garlic, dried dill, salt, and pepper in a bowl.

4. Pour the mixture over the cod fillets.

5. Bake for 15-20 minutes or until fish flakes easily.

6. Garnish with lemon wedges before serving.

Nutritional Value: Calories: 180 | Protein: 24g | Carbohydrates: 2g | Fiber: 0g | Fat: 8g

Recipe 49: Berry and Chia Seed Smoothie

Prep Time: 10 minutes

Ingredients:

- 1 cup mixed berries (strawberries, blueberries, raspberries)
- 1 cup almond milk
- 2 tablespoons chia seeds
- 1 tablespoon honey (optional)
- Ice cubes (optional)

Directions:

1. Blend mixed berries and almond milk until smooth.
2. Add chia seeds and honey, blend again.
3. Add ice cubes if desired.

Nutritional Value: Calories: 200 | Protein: 4g | Carbohydrates: 30g | Fiber: 11g | Fat: 7g

Recipe 50: Mediterranean Stuffed Bell Peppers

Prep Time: 45 minutes

Ingredients:

- 4 bell peppers, any color
- 1 cup cooked quinoa
- 1/2 cup diced tomatoes
- 1/2 cup diced cucumber
- 1/4 cup Kalamata olives, sliced

- 1/4 cup crumbled feta cheese
- 2 tablespoons fresh parsley, chopped
- 2 tablespoons olive oil
- Juice of 1 lemon

Directions:

1. Preheat oven to 375°F (190°C).
2. Cut the tops off the bell peppers and remove the seeds and membranes.
3. In a bowl, mix cooked quinoa, diced tomatoes, diced cucumber, sliced Kalamata olives, crumbled feta cheese, chopped fresh parsley, olive oil, lemon juice, salt, and pepper.
4. Stuff each bell pepper with the quinoa mixture.
5. Place stuffed peppers in a baking dish, cover with foil, and bake for 25-30 minutes until peppers are tender.

Nutritional Value:

Calories: 250 | Protein: 7g | Carbohydrates: 28g | Fiber: 6g | Fat: 13g

Recipe 51: Cilantro and Lime Rice

Prep Time: 15 minutes

Ingredients:

- 1 cup long-grain white rice

- 2 cups water

- 1/4 cup fresh cilantro, chopped

- Juice of 1 lime

- Salt to taste

Directions:

1. Rinse rice under cold water until the water runs clear.

2. In a saucepan, combine rice and water. Bring to a boil, then reduce heat to low, cover, and simmer for 15-20 minutes or until rice is tender.

3. Fluff the cooked rice with a fork.

4. Stir in chopped cilantro, lime juice, and salt.

Nutritional Value: Calories: 200 | Protein: 4g | Carbohydrates: 45g | Fiber: 1g | Fat: 0g

Recipe 52: Turmeric and Cumin Roasted Cauliflower

Prep Time: 25 minutes

Ingredients:

- 1 head cauliflower, cut into florets

- 2 tablespoons olive oil

- 1 teaspoon turmeric powder

- 1 teaspoon ground cumin

- Salt and pepper to taste

Directions:

1. Preheat oven to 425°F (220°C).

2. Toss cauliflower florets with olive oil, turmeric powder, ground cumin, salt, and pepper.

3. Spread in a single layer on a baking sheet.

4. Roast for 20-25 minutes or until cauliflower is golden and tender.

Nutritional Value: Calories: 100 | Protein: 3g | Carbohydrates: 9g | Fiber: 3g | Fat: 7g

Recipe 53: Blueberry and Spinach Smoothie

Prep Time: 10 minutes

Ingredients:

- 1 cup fresh spinach leaves

- 1/2 cup blueberries

- 1/2 banana

- 1/2 cup Greek yogurt

- 1/2 cup almond milk

- 1 tablespoon honey (optional)

- Ice cubes (optional)

Directions:

1. Blend spinach leaves, blueberries, banana, Greek yogurt, almond milk, and honey until smooth.

2. Add ice cubes if desired.

Nutritional Value: Calories: 180 | Protein: 8g | Carbohydrates: 30g | Fiber: 5g | Fat: 3g

Recipe 54: Roasted Garlic and Herb Asparagus

Prep Time: 20 minutes

Ingredients:

- 1 bunch asparagus, trimmed

- 2 tablespoons olive oil

- 4 cloves garlic, minced

- 2 tablespoons fresh herbs (rosemary, thyme, or parsley), chopped

- Salt and pepper to taste

- Lemon wedges for garnish

Directions:

1. Preheat oven to 400°F (200°C).

2. Toss asparagus with olive oil, minced garlic, fresh herbs, salt, and pepper.

3. Roast for 12-15 minutes or until asparagus is tender.

4. Garnish with lemon wedges before serving.

Nutritional Value: Calories: 90 | Protein: 3g | Carbohydrates: 5g | Fiber: 2g | Fat: 7g

Recipe 55: Mango and Turmeric Lassi

Prep Time: 10 minutes

Ingredients:

- 1 ripe mango, peeled and diced

- 1 cup plain yogurt

- 1/2 cup almond milk

- 1/2 teaspoon turmeric powder

- 1 tablespoon honey (optional)

- Pinch of cardamom (optional)

- Ice cubes (optional)

Directions:

1. Blend diced mango, plain yogurt, almond milk, turmeric powder, and honey until smooth.

2. Add a pinch of cardamom and ice cubes if desired.

Nutritional Value: Calories: 150 | Protein: 4g | Carbohydrates: 28g | Fiber: 3g | Fat: 4g

Recipe 56: Balsamic Glazed Brussels Sprouts

Prep Time: 30 minutes

Ingredients:

- 1 pound Brussels sprouts, trimmed and halved

- 2 tablespoons olive oil

- 2 tablespoons balsamic vinegar

- 1 tablespoon honey

- Salt and pepper to taste

Directions:

1. Preheat oven to 400°F (200°C).

2. Toss Brussels sprouts with olive oil, balsamic vinegar, honey, salt, and pepper.

3. Roast for 20-25 minutes or until tender and caramelized.

Nutritional Value: Calories: 120 | Protein: 3g | Carbohydrates: 15g | Fiber: 4g | Fat: 6g

Recipe 57: Avocado and Tomato Salad

Prep Time: 10 minutes

Ingredients:

- 2 ripe avocados, diced

- 2 tomatoes, diced

- 1/4 cup red onion, finely chopped

- 2 tablespoons fresh cilantro, chopped

- Juice of 1 lime

- Salt and pepper to taste

Directions:

1. In a bowl, combine diced avocados, diced tomatoes, finely chopped red onion, chopped fresh cilantro, lime juice, salt, and pepper.

2. Gently toss to combine.

Nutritional Value: Calories: 200 | Protein: 3g | Carbohydrates: 15g | Fiber: 8g | Fat: 16g

Recipe 58: Quinoa and Black Bean Stuffed Peppers

Prep Time: 45 minutes

Ingredients:

- 4 bell peppers, any color

- 1 cup cooked quinoa

- 1 cup black beans, cooked and drained

- 1/2 cup corn kernels

- 1/2 cup diced tomatoes

- 1/4 cup red onion, finely chopped

- 2 tablespoons taco seasoning

- Salt and pepper to taste

- Shredded cheddar cheese (optional)

Directions:

1. Preheat oven to 375°F (190°C).

2. Cut the tops off the bell peppers and remove the seeds and membranes.

3. In a bowl, mix cooked quinoa, black beans, corn kernels, diced tomatoes, finely chopped red onion, taco seasoning, salt, and pepper.

4. Stuff each bell pepper with the quinoa mixture.

5. Place stuffed peppers in a baking dish, cover with foil, and bake for 25-30 minutes until peppers are tender.

6. If desired, top with shredded cheddar cheese and bake for an additional 5 minutes until cheese is melted.

Nutritional Value: Calories: 300 | Protein: 10g | Carbohydrates: 55g | Fiber: 10g | Fat: 5g

Recipe 59: Paprika and Garlic Shrimp

Prep Time: 20 minutes

Ingredients:

- 1 pound large shrimp, peeled and deveined

- 2 tablespoons olive oil

- 2 cloves garlic, minced

- 1 teaspoon smoked paprika

- Juice of 1 lemon

- Fresh parsley for garnish

- Salt and pepper to taste

Directions:

1. In a bowl, mix shrimp with olive oil, minced garlic, smoked paprika, lemon juice, salt, and pepper.

2. Heat a skillet over medium-high heat.

3. Cook shrimp for 2-3 minutes per side or until pink and opaque.

4. Garnish with fresh parsley before serving.

Nutritional Value: Calories: 180 | Protein: 22g | Carbohydrates: 2g | Fiber: 0g | Fat: 9g

Recipe 60: Greek Yogurt Parfait with Berries

Prep Time: 10 minutes

Ingredients:

- 1 cup Greek yogurt

- 1/2 cup mixed berries (strawberries, blueberries, raspberries)

- 1/4 cup granola

- 1 tablespoon honey (optional)

Directions:

1. In a glass or bowl, layer Greek yogurt, mixed berries, granola, and drizzle with honey if desired.

Nutritional Value: Calories: 280 | Protein: 15g | Carbohydrates: 40g | Fiber: 5g | Fat: 8g

CONCLUSION

As we reach the end of "Thyroid-Healing Recipes for Hormone Balance: Nourishing Your Body, Restoring Your Vitality," we want to express our heartfelt gratitude for joining us on this culinary adventure. We hope that this cookbook has not only filled your kitchen with delicious aromas and flavors but has also provided you with valuable tools to support your thyroid health and hormonal balance.

Our aim was to create a collection of recipes that not only taste incredible but also contribute to your overall well-being. A healthy thyroid is a cornerstone of vitality, and these recipes are designed to nourish and support this vital gland.

We encourage you to continue exploring the world of thyroid-friendly cuisine, experimenting with ingredients, and enjoying the benefits of a balanced diet. Remember that your journey to better health and hormone balance is unique to you, and the choices you make in the kitchen can have a profound impact on your quality of life.

In this cookbook, we've shared recipes that range from quick and easy weekday meals to special occasions, ensuring that you have a variety of options to suit your lifestyle and dietary preferences. We've also included nutritional information for each recipe, empowering you to make informed choices about the foods you consume.

Please don't hesitate to revisit these recipes whenever you seek nourishment, comfort, or a boost to your thyroid health. We believe that food can be a powerful source of healing, and each meal you prepare from this cookbook is a step towards a healthier, more balanced you.

Thank you for choosing to prioritize your health and well-being through the art of cooking. We hope these recipes have brought joy to your kitchen and have set you on a path to greater vitality and harmony within your body.